Book Title: "Surviving the Shadows: Confronting Salmonella" **Bowel Obstruction Symptoms Bowel Obstruction Symptoms Scleroderma Symptoms**

Chapter Titles:

Book Introduction

In the darkness of the invisible, there lurks a treacherous adversary: Salmonella. A cunning bacterium that strikes unexpectedly, it is responsible for countless illnesses and even deaths worldwide. Its enigmatic nature has haunted scientists and doctors for centuries, leaving behind a trail of fear and uncertainty.

In "Surviving the Shadows: Confronting Salmonella," we embark on a journey to uncover the secrets of this elusive foe. Guided by the light of knowledge, we'll reveal its origins, how it infiltrates our bodies, and the devastating toll it takes on human health.

Beyond the clinical facts, this book aims to touch your heart and stir your emotions. It is not merely a scientific account but a testament to the courage of those who have faced this shadowy enemy and survived. Their stories resonate through these pages, inspiring us to confront our fears and stand resilient against the darkness that seeks to engulf us.

Throughout this emotional exploration, we'll learn about the symptoms that torment victims, the unsuspecting carriers who unknowingly spread the contagion, and the common sources where the bacterium hides. We'll delve into the food industry's challenges and the vulnerabilities of certain populations in their fight against Salmonella.

As we journey together, we'll also uncover the efforts of brave souls who have dedicated their lives to investigating and battling this insidious invader. From epidemiologists on the trail of outbreaks to researchers developing innovative solutions, we will witness the relentless pursuit of a safer world.

"Surviving the Shadows: Confronting Salmonella" is not only a tale of woe but a beacon of hope. It empowers us with knowledge, equipping us to defend ourselves and our loved ones from this formidable adversary. Join me as we confront our fears and walk through the darkness, guided by the light of understanding, unity, and compassion.

Chapter 1: Unseen Threats: Understanding Salmonella

Within the hidden realm of microorganisms, Salmonella lurks as a formidable menace, affecting millions across the globe. This chapter unveils the enigma surrounding this bacterium, exploring its history, characteristics, and the numerous serotypes that plague humanity. As we delve into the scientific intricacies, we'll witness the emotional and physical toll it takes on those unfortunate enough to cross paths with this unseen enemy.

Salmonella's journey begins, as we venture back through time, tracing its discovery and the scientific breakthroughs that have led to our current understanding of its pathogenicity. We'll explore the diverse serotypes, each with its unique traits and capabilities, revealing the complexities that challenge researchers and healthcare professionals alike.

But this chapter is not solely a scientific exposé; it delves into the human side of the story. We'll hear firsthand accounts from individuals who have experienced the torment of Salmonella infection, their struggles, fears, and ultimately, their triumphs over this relentless foe.

As we uncover the emotional aspects, we'll also discuss the common symptoms that assail those infected. From the mild discomfort that rattles daily routines to the severe manifestations that threaten lives, the breadth of Salmonella's impact becomes evident.

Join me on this emotional journey as we unravel the mysteries surrounding Salmonella, understanding its origins and discovering the unyielding spirit of those who have confronted and survived this unseen threat. Together, we shall find the strength to face the shadows and emerge victorious against this ancient and ruthless adversary.

Chapter 1 Continued...

Unseen Threats: Understanding Salmonella

In the dark corners of the scientific world, where mysteries abound, a tiny, malevolent organism silently thrives—Salmonella. Its name might sound innocuous, but the havoc it wreaks upon the human body is anything but benign. As we delve further into the depths of this chapter, brace yourself for the emotional rollercoaster that awaits, as stories of pain, resilience, and courage unfold.

Imagine a young mother, holding her feverish child close, the worry etched deeply in her eyes as she watches the innocent life she brought into the world suffer at the hands of an invisible enemy. Picture the elderly, whose golden years should be filled with laughter and joy, instead tormented by a relentless illness that steals away their strength and independence. These heart-wrenching scenes play out daily across the world, a stark reminder of the insidious nature of Salmonella.

But in the face of adversity, hope emerges. Within the annals of medical history, there are tales of triumph over this dreaded pathogen—of ordinary individuals displaying extraordinary resilience. These are the stories that will inspire you to stand strong, to be vigilant, and to take action.

As we explore the origins of Salmonella, you'll come to understand that this is not just a story of bacteria and disease. It is a narrative that binds us all together, uniting us in a shared struggle against a common enemy. From the bustling cities to the remotest corners of the earth, no one is immune to its reach.

Throughout history, scientists have waged a tireless war against this invisible foe. Pioneering research has illuminated the path to understanding Salmonella's inner workings, but there is still much to be learned. As we embark on this emotional journey, we'll come to appreciate the dedication and sacrifice of those who dedicate their lives to this crucial cause.

The symptoms of Salmonella infection vary, ranging from stomach cramps and diarrhea to severe dehydration and life-threatening complications. For some, the battle is short-lived, but for others, it becomes a lifelong struggle, leaving lasting physical and emotional scars.

Let us not forget those who remain silent carriers, unknowingly spreading the infection to vulnerable populations. This chapter will confront the harsh realities and moral dilemmas faced by these unwitting culprits, reminding us that compassion and understanding are essential in the quest to eradicate Salmonella.

In "Unseen Threats: Understanding Salmonella," we have embarked on a voyage through time and emotion, where the triumphs and tragedies of countless souls converge. Let the depths of this exploration move you, instilling a sense of urgency to protect yourself and your loved ones.

Knowledge is our most potent weapon against this shadowy adversary. Armed with the insights gained from this chapter, we can better comprehend the magnitude of the threat we face and take the first steps towards safeguarding our communities.

In the forthcoming chapters, we will unveil more layers of this poignant tale—peering into the battlegrounds of the human body, investigating the sources of contamination, and discovering the heroes who strive tirelessly to bring light to the darkest corners of this microbial world.

Stay with me, dear reader, as we continue this expedition together. Our emotions may be stirred, but our resolve will be strengthened, for it is in unity that we find the strength to confront the unseen threats and emerge victorious over Salmonella.

Chapter 2: The Insidious Invader: How Salmonella Infects

In the deepest recesses of our bodies, a silent invasion takes place—one that leaves devastation in its wake. This chapter unravels the chilling mechanisms by which Salmonella infiltrates our defenses, leaving us vulnerable to its malevolence. Brace yourself, for we are about to embark on an emotional journey into the microscopic battleground where life and death collide.

Imagine the moment when a seemingly innocuous meal becomes a harbinger of suffering. The joy of sharing a delicious feast with loved ones turns into a nightmare, as the enemy cunningly finds its way onto the plate, camouflaged within the very sustenance meant to nourish us. This insidious invader knows no bounds, sparing no one in its pursuit of a host.

In this chapter, we'll delve into the tactics employed by Salmonella to breach our body's fortress. From the moment it sets foot within our system, it launches a relentless assault, seeking to establish a stronghold from which to wreak havoc. The emotional intensity escalates as we witness the battle at the cellular level—the struggle for supremacy between pathogen and immune cells.

Even more harrowing are the stories of those whose bodies bear the scars of past confrontations with Salmonella. Their voices echo through the pages, recounting the agony of symptoms that seemingly never end, the frustration of recurrent infections, and the fear that lingers long after the bacterium has been vanquished.

As we navigate this emotional labyrinth, we'll uncover the vulnerable populations—the innocent victims caught in the crossfire of this microscopic war. The elderly, whose weakened defenses provide an entry point for the enemy; the children, whose tiny bodies fight valiantly against an unseen adversary; and the immunocompromised, who are forced to endure a constant state of vigilance.

In the face of such malevolence, hope flickers like a distant candle. But it is not extinguished. Medical professionals and researchers stand at the forefront, waging a tireless battle against the insidious invader. We'll encounter their stories of determination, of the sleepless nights spent in the pursuit of knowledge, and of the moments of triumph that spur them on.

Yet, amidst the scientific revelations, we must not lose sight of the emotional toll this relentless struggle extracts from its victims. The psychological scars left behind, the anxiety that lingers, and the sense of vulnerability that remains—these are the emotional footprints that Salmonella leaves behind.

In the labyrinth of this chapter, we come face to face with the stark reality that we are not alone in this fight.

Every soul touched by Salmonella's malevolence is part of a collective struggle—a global narrative that demands our attention and empathy.

Dear reader, as we journey deeper into the intricate world of Salmonella, let us not become numb to the emotional gravity of this battle. For in understanding the emotional landscape, we forge a connection—a bond that unites us in solidarity against a common foe.

With each revelation, with each personal account, we are stirred to confront the insidious invader with renewed vigor. Let compassion be our shield, and knowledge our s, as we strive to protect ourselves and those we hold dear from the clutches of this microscopic menace.

Continue to walk beside me as we traverse this emotional terrain. The path ahead may be arduous, but together, we can unravel the mysteries of Salmonella and take one step closer to unmasking the hidden enemy within.

Chapter 3: Battling the Beast Within: Body's Fight Against Salmonella

In the arena of life, a fierce battle unfolds every time Salmonella gains entry into the body. This chapter illuminates the valiant efforts of our immune system as it wages war against the invader. Through tears of pain and triumph, we witness the indomitable spirit of the human body, fighting to reclaim its territory from the relentless beast within.

Picture the body as a battlefield, where the courageous defenders—the immune cells—marshal their forces to confront the malevolent intruder. It is a scene of chaos and order, where every move and countermove is calculated, and where the stakes are nothing short of life and death.

In this emotional journey, we'll encounter the tales of brave souls who have faced the onslaught of Salmonella and lived to tell their story. Each one is a testament to the strength and resilience of the human spirit. They fought fever and chills, endured the relentless assault on their digestive system, and emerged scarred but victorious from the battlefield.

As we dive deeper, we'll come to appreciate the intricacies of the immune system—the elegant dance of white blood cells, antibodies, and cytokines that orchestrate a symphony of defense. Witness the surge of emotions that engulf a patient when their body begins to rally against the invader, providing a glimmer of hope amidst the darkness of illness.

However, in the face of a formidable foe like Salmonella, victory is not guaranteed. For some, the battle takes an agonizing turn, as the immune system struggles to contain the relentless assault. We'll confront the harsh reality of severe infections and the emotional toll it exacts on both the afflicted and their loved ones.

But even in the darkest moments, there are glimpses of light—stories of courage and determination that leave us in awe. The medical professionals who tirelessly stand at the frontline, guiding patients through the storm with unwavering compassion and expertise, are the unsung heroes of this battle.

This chapter isn't just a scientific account of cellular warfare; it is an emotional exploration of the human spirit, tenacious in its struggle against an unseen adversary. The tears shed in pain are mirrored by tears of joy when a patient triumphantly emerges from the clutches of illness, grateful for another chance at life.

As we navigate the emotional landscape of this chapter, we must also acknowledge the toll on mental health. The fear of the unknown, the uncertainty of the outcome, and the vulnerability felt during illness—we must confront these emotional scars and provide support to those who bear them.

In the end, it is not just the physical body that fights against Salmonella, but the heart and soul of the individual. Each battle fought, whether won or lost, leaves an indelible mark—a reminder of the human spirit's strength in the face of adversity.

Dear reader, be prepared to experience the full gamut of emotions as we bear witness to the triumphs and tribulations of the human body's fight against the relentless beast within. Together, we'll gain a deeper appreciation for the fragility and resilience of life, and find solace in the knowledge that we are not alone in this battle.

Let us forge ahead with empathy and understanding, and may the stories in this chapter stir our souls to be more compassionate, more resilient, and more united in our quest to conquer the beast within and emerge victorious against the clutches of Salmonella.

Chapter 4: The Silent Danger: Asymptomatic Carriers of Salmonella

Beyond the obvious symptoms and visible suffering, there exists a concealed threat that quietly perpetuates the cycle of infection—silent carriers of Salmonella. This chapter explores the enigmatic world of those who unknowingly bear the burden of this insidious bacterium, casting an emotional spotlight on the complexities of transmission and the moral dilemmas they face.

Imagine a seemingly healthy individual, blissfully unaware of the danger they pose to others. They move through life, their daily routines and interactions unwittingly becoming potential vectors of Salmonella transmission. The silent danger lies in the fact that these carriers, devoid of symptoms themselves, unwittingly become the catalysts for outbreaks that ripple through communities.

In this chapter, we will encounter the stories of those who have inadvertently become conduits of infection. Their emotions are a swirling tempest, oscillating between guilt and innocence, as they grapple with the burden of being the unknowing spreaders of a hidden danger.

It is within the hearts of these carriers that we find the complex intersection of individual responsibility and societal impact. Their emotional journey is one of conflicting emotions—fear of judgment and remorse for the harm they might unknowingly cause.

But let us not be hasty in passing judgment, for the emotional turmoil experienced by these carriers is not to be underestimated. The knowledge that their actions, however innocuous, might inadvertently lead to suffering for others is a heavy weight to bear.

As we immerse ourselves in the emotional depths of this chapter, we are reminded that empathy and understanding are vital in our collective effort to combat Salmonella. The silent carriers are among us, interwoven in the fabric of our communities, and it is only through unity and compassion that we can hope to break the chains of transmission.

This chapter also underscores the importance of vigilance in identifying and tracing asymptomatic carriers. Medical professionals and public health authorities become the detectives in this narrative, navigating the delicate balance between privacy and the greater good. Their emotional journey is one of perseverance and resilience as they work tirelessly to protect communities from the silent danger that lurks in the shadows.

Let us, as compassionate readers, not turn a blind eye to the emotional plight of these silent carriers. Instead, let their stories serve as a call to action—a plea for increased awareness, improved testing, and robust contact tracing. Together, we can create a safer environment for everyone, where the burden of silent transmission is lifted from the shoulders of unsuspecting carriers.

As we traverse the emotional landscape of this chapter, we will come to understand that addressing the silent danger of asymptomatic carriers requires a delicate dance—one that balances individual rights with the collective wellbeing. It is a testament to our shared humanity that we strive to protect both ourselves and others, forging an unbreakable bond that transcends borders and boundaries.

Dear reader, as you journey through this chapter, may you be moved by the emotional intricacies that underpin the world of silent carriers. Let empathy guide your steps as we unite to confront the hidden threats of Salmonella, and may the resilience of the human spirit inspire us to forge a future where the silent danger is silenced, and our communities stand stronger together.

Chapter 5: Unmasking the Culprits: Common Sources of Salmonella Contamination

The search for the shadowy origins of Salmonella takes us on a heart-wrenching expedition through the common sources of contamination. In this chapter, emotions will run high as we unmask the unsuspecting culprits—the very elements we once trusted to nourish and sustain us. Brace yourself, as we confront the harsh reality that the enemy might be lurking in the most unexpected places.

Picture the vibrant marketplace, where colorful fruits and vegetables entice passersby with promises of health and vitality. Yet, beneath their alluring façade, lies the potential threat of Salmonella, waiting to strike the unwary. The emotional turmoil surfaces as we grapple with the realization that the culprits might be hiding in plain sight.

In this emotional journey, we'll explore the food industry—a complex web of growers, processors, and distributors. Their struggle to balance profits with safety becomes a battle of conscience, as they confront the ethical implications of potentially endangering consumers through inadvertent contamination.

Our hearts will ache for the devoted farmers, whose toil under the scorching sun is rewarded with bountiful harvests. But even the most diligent among them can unknowingly become victims of this relentless enemy. Their anguish is real, as they stand torn between their livelihood and the potential risks to public health.

In our quest to unmask the culprits, we'll encounter the emotional narratives of foodborne illness victims. The moments of joy and celebration shattered by the anguish of illness—these are the stories that will stay with us long after this chapter's end. Their voices serve as a poignant reminder that the battle against Salmonella is not waged in isolation; it is a collective struggle that unites us all.

At the heart of this chapter lies the need for accountability. Food safety is a shared responsibility—a pact between producers and consumers. We must be vigilant in demanding transparency and safety measures from the food industry while taking the necessary precautions in our own homes.

Medical professionals, too, play a crucial role in unmasking the culprits. With compassion and empathy, they work to diagnose and treat those affected by Salmonella-contaminated food. Their dedication and emotional investment in the well-being of their patients inspire us to seek justice and prevention.

In our pursuit of understanding, we must also acknowledge the emotional toll borne by those in the food industry. The weight of responsibility they carry is immense, as they strive to maintain high standards while navigating the complexities of a globalized market.

As we navigate the emotional depths of this chapter, may our hearts be filled with resolve—to stand firm in the face of deception and demand the highest standards of food safety. Let us honor the stories of victims and survivors alike by working together to unmask the culprits and create a safer, more transparent food landscape.

Dear reader, the emotional impact of this chapter serves as a call to action—a reminder that the battle against Salmonella requires vigilance, compassion, and collective effort. The common sources of contamination are within our grasp, and with determination and unity, we can unravel the mystery and emerge triumphant in our quest to protect ourselves and our loved ones.

Continue with me, as we journey further into the labyrinth of Salmonella's world. Embrace the emotions that arise, for it is through this emotional connection that we find the strength to unmask the culprits and forge a path towards a safer, healthier future for all.

Chapter 6: A Culinary Hazard: Salmonella in Food Products

In the heart of our homes and kitchens lies a double-edged s—food, the source of sustenance and joy, can also harbor a hidden hazard—Salmonella. This chapter delves into the emotional complexities of our culinary haven, where the simple act of nourishment becomes a precarious dance with danger. Prepare to confront your emotions, for the battle against Salmonella takes on a deeply personal tone within these walls.

Imagine the joy of cooking for loved ones, the aroma of home-cooked meals filling the air, and the anticipation of shared laughter around the dinner table. Yet, amidst this idyllic scene, lurks the emotional turmoil of uncertainty. Is the food we've lovingly prepared truly safe Can we protect our families from an unseen enemy that defies the senses

This chapter invites us to witness the emotional journey of home cooks and chefs alike—the guardians of our culinary havens. Their passion for creating culinary delights is matched only by their commitment to food safety. The weight of responsibility they carry is palpable, as they navigate the delicate balance between culinary artistry and the need to safeguard against contamination.

In the aftermath of a foodborne illness outbreak, emotions run high as investigations unfold. The guilt that washes over those in the food industry is profound, as they grapple with the realization that their creations might have inadvertently caused harm.

For the victims of Salmonella-contaminated food, the emotional scars run deep. The dining table, once a place of comfort and nourishment, becomes a symbol of fear and uncertainty. These are the stories that tug at our heartstrings, urging us to be vigilant in safeguarding our food supply and demanding accountability.

But amidst the darkness, rays of hope emerge. This chapter celebrates the unwavering commitment of food safety advocates and regulatory bodies, who labor behind the scenes to protect consumers. Their emotional investment in public health serves as a beacon of light in the fight against this culinary hazard.

As we explore the emotional landscape of this chapter, we must also reckon with the reality that we, as consumers, play a vital role in this battle. The choices we make in the grocery store and the precautions we take in our kitchens can make a world of difference. Let us be driven by the desire to protect our families and our communities, to transform our dining spaces into sanctuaries of safety.

Medical professionals are not exempt from this narrative, as they stand ready to diagnose and treat those affected by foodborne illness. Their compassion and dedication inspire us to seek better systems, where early detection and swift action can prevent further harm.

Dear reader, as we journey deeper into the culinary landscape of Salmonella, let us be moved by the emotional undercurrents that bind us to our food. May we approach our kitchens with mindfulness and caution, and may the emotional narratives within this chapter empower us to be proactive in the fight against this hidden menace.

Continue with me, as we shed light on the dark corners of Salmonella's culinary domain. Let empathy guide our steps as we navigate the emotional intricacies of this chapter, and may the shared desire for safer food unite us in a resolute pursuit of a future where our meals are not just delicious, but also free from the threat of contamination.

Chapter 7: The Hidden Outbreak: Salmonella in Water and Environment

In the vast expanse of nature and the very water that sustains life, lurks an insidious presence—Salmonella. This chapter delves into the emotional dimensions of this hidden outbreak, where the elements we rely on for survival become potential sources of contamination. Brace yourself for an emotional exploration of our connection to the environment and the urgent need to protect the precious resources that sustain us.

Imagine the soothing sound of a babbling brook, the sense of wonder as raindrops kiss the earth, and the tranquility of a pristine lake. Nature's beauty provides solace to our weary souls, but within this idyllic setting, danger looms. The emotional paradox arises as we come to terms with the realization that even the purest of sources can harbor the threat of Salmonella.

In this chapter, we'll follow the emotional journeys of environmental experts and conservationists. Their mission to safeguard the earth's natural resources is both inspiring and daunting. They face the challenge of balancing humanity's needs with the preservation of ecosystems, all while combatting the risk of Salmonella contamination.

As we delve deeper, we'll encounter the emotional turmoil experienced by communities affected by environmental outbreaks. The very land they call home, and the water they rely on for sustenance, becomes a source of fear and uncertainty. We'll bear witness to their struggles, their resilience, and their calls for urgent action to protect their health and that of future generations.

Yet, amidst the shadows, there are rays of hope. This chapter celebrates the efforts of dedicated researchers, who tirelessly investigate the sources of environmental contamination. Their emotional investment in unraveling the mysteries of Salmonella in water and nature fuels our shared quest for knowledge and action.

But the burden of responsibility does not rest solely on scientists and environmentalists. Each of us has a role to play in safeguarding the environment and our water sources. The emotional weight of this reality is a call to action —a plea to cherish and protect the very resources that sustain us.

Medical professionals, too, find themselves entwined in the narrative of the hidden outbreak. As they treat patients affected by waterborne Salmonella, their hearts are heavy with the knowledge that prevention is the ultimate cure.

Dear reader, as we navigate the emotional depths of this chapter, may our hearts be filled with a profound appreciation for the interconnectedness of life. The hidden outbreak reminds us that our actions have consequences, not just for ourselves but for the entire web of existence.

Let us rise together, as stewards of the earth, and recognize that our fates are inextricably tied to the health of our environment. The emotional narratives within this chapter call upon us to embrace sustainability, advocate for conservation, and strive for a future where nature's beauty and the water that sustains us remain pure and untainted.

Continue with me, as we uncover the hidden truths lurking in the waters and the environment. Let empathy guide our steps, and may the emotional revelations propel us towards collective action—a shared mission to protect the delicate balance of our planet and ensure a safer, healthier world for generations to come.

Chapter 8: A Risky Business: Salmonella in the Food Industry

Amidst the bustling factories and frenetic kitchens, the food industry emerges as a complex battleground against Salmonella. This chapter delves into the emotional undercurrents of a risky business—where profit and safety collide, and the human cost of contamination becomes all too real. Prepare to confront the raw emotions of those entwined in this industry, as they navigate the delicate dance between commerce and the wellbeing of consumers.

Picture the assembly lines in motion, churning out products destined for millions of plates. It is a world of efficiency and productivity, where the bottom line reigns supreme. Yet, within this mechanized process, lies the risk—the potential for Salmonella to infiltrate the very sustenance that nourishes us.

In this emotional journey, we'll encounter the stories of those who toil behind the scenes—the factory workers, the food handlers, and the farmers. Their livelihoods are entwined with the food they produce, and the weight of responsibility they bear is immense. The emotional toll of ensuring food safety while meeting commercial demands is a balancing act that requires superhuman resilience.

For those who have witnessed foodborne illness outbreaks linked to their products, the emotional scars run deep. The heartache of knowing that their hard work might have unwittingly caused harm to consumers becomes an emotional burden that cannot be easily shrugged off.

As we navigate the intricacies of this chapter, we must also confront the harsh reality of profit-driven decision-making. The pressure to meet demand, to cut costs, and to optimize processes can sometimes overshadow the importance of ensuring food safety.

But in this risky business, heroes emerge—food safety professionals who serve as the guardians of the food industry. Their emotional investment in protecting consumers is unwavering, as they work tirelessly to implement and enforce safety measures that can save lives.

The emotional journeys of these professionals, entwined with those of medical experts, collide when outbreaks occur. Both groups are united by a shared purpose—to protect public health and prevent further harm. Their dedication is an inspiring testament to the human spirit's capacity for compassion and resilience.

Dear reader, as we delve deeper into the risky business of the food industry, let us be moved by the emotional narratives that underpin this world. Let empathy guide our understanding of the challenges faced by those in the industry, and let compassion inspire us to demand accountability for food safety.

In this chapter, we bear witness to the complexity of the food industry's landscape—a world where commerce and consumer safety intersect. Let us be driven by the emotional investment of those who strive for a safer future—a future where our meals are not just delectable but also free from the hidden danger of Salmonella.

Continue with me, as we navigate the emotional labyrinth of this chapter. May the stories we encounter stir our souls to advocate for transparency, accountability, and the collective responsibility to prioritize the wellbeing of consumers over all else. Together, we can transform this risky business into a resolute pursuit of a safer and more compassionate food industry.

Chapter 9: Vulnerable Populations: Children, Elderly, and Immunocompromised

Within the tapestry of humanity, there exist those who are most vulnerable—the children, the elderly, and the immunocompromised. This chapter delves into the emotional depths of their plight, as they face the heightened risks posed by Salmonella. Prepare to be moved by their stories of courage, resilience, and the collective responsibility to protect those who are most fragile among us.

Imagine the innocent laughter of children, their bright eyes brimming with wonder, and their tender bodies still developing defenses against the world's dangers. It is in these tiny souls that the emotional weight of vulnerability becomes palpable. Our hearts ache as we confront the reality that the innocent are often the most affected by the relentless assault of Salmonella.

This chapter also takes us to the twilight of life—the realm of the elderly, who have weathered life's storms and now seek solace in their golden years. But as age sets in, so does frailty, and the emotional complexity arises when the twilight years are tainted by the shadow of illness.

And then, there are the immunocompromised—the warriors whose immune systems are already engaged in other battles. For them, the presence of Salmonella becomes a formidable foe, an additional burden that their already weakened bodies must bear.

In this emotional journey, we'll encounter the stories of caregivers—the unsung heroes who stand as pillars of strength for the vulnerable. Their dedication to safeguarding those in their care is an emotional investment that knows no bounds. Their love is a balm for wounds, and their support becomes a lifeline for those facing the odds.

As we navigate this chapter's emotional labyrinth, we must confront the harsh reality that those we hold dear—our children, our elders, and our immunocompromised loved ones—are the most susceptible to the clutches of Salmonella. This knowledge becomes a catalyst for collective action—to protect the vulnerable and ensure that they are shielded from harm.

Medical professionals dedicated to caring for these populations bear the weight of immense responsibility. Their emotional connection with their patients is a guiding force, as they seek to provide the best possible care and advocate for prevention.

Dear reader, as we journey deeper into the vulnerability of these precious lives, let us be moved to compassion and empathy. The emotional narratives of children, elderly, and immunocompromised individuals call upon us to be their voices—to stand united in a resolute mission to protect those who need us most.

Let us be driven by the love in our hearts—the love that compels us to act, to demand better systems, and to create a world where the vulnerable are shielded from harm. Together, we can be the guardians of the innocent, the protectors of the twilight years, and the advocates for those whose immune systems need a helping hand.

Continue with me, dear reader, as we delve further into the vulnerability of these cherished souls. May the emotional connections we forge fuel our collective determination to create a world where the vulnerable are embraced, safeguarded, and cherished with the love and compassion they truly deserve.

Chapter 10: Light in the Darkness: Triumphs and Hope Against Salmonella

In the shadows cast by the relentless threat of Salmonella, rays of light break through—triumphs, courage, and hope illuminate the path forward. This chapter celebrates the emotional victories won against the bacterium and the relentless spirit of those who refuse to succumb to fear. Prepare to be inspired, as we bear witness to the human capacity to rise above adversity and find hope in the face of darkness.

Imagine the jubilation of a recovered patient, the joyous embrace of a family reunited after illness, and the tears of relief shed by caregivers. These emotional moments of triumph are the heart of this chapter, for they remind us that amidst the darkness of illness, hope shines like a beacon.

In this emotional journey, we'll encounter the stories of survivors—ordinary individuals who displayed extraordinary resilience in their battle against Salmonella. Their emotional strength is a testament to the human spirit's ability to endure and overcome, and their stories serve as beacons of hope for others facing the same fight.

As we delve deeper into the emotional victories, we must also recognize the tireless efforts of medical professionals and researchers. Their commitment to advancing knowledge and developing new treatments is a source of hope for the future—a future where Salmonella's hold on humanity is weakened.

This chapter is also an homage to the unsung heroes—the individuals and organizations dedicated to food safety, environmental protection, and public health. Their emotional investment in safeguarding communities shines through as they work tirelessly to prevent further harm.

The emotional journey of triumph is not without its challenges, as setbacks and hurdles can dampen spirits. But amidst the storm, hope persists. It is a beacon that guides us through the darkness, reminding us that with each victory, we draw closer to a safer, healthier world.

Dear reader, as we embrace the emotional triumphs within this chapter, let us be moved to see the hope that exists within each of us. The victories against Salmonella are not confined to laboratories or hospitals—they are woven into the very fabric of humanity.

Let us be inspired by the courage of survivors, the dedication of medical professionals, and the passion of food safety advocates. Their emotional journeys remind us that we are not passive observers in the fight against Salmonella—we are active participants, united in our pursuit of a brighter, healthier future.

Continue with me, as we navigate the emotional tapestry of triumph and hope. May the stories within this chapter ignite a flame within our hearts —a flame of determination and optimism, as we forge ahead with renewed resolve to conquer Salmonella and embrace the light in the darkness.

Chapter 11: A Call to Unity: Forging Bonds Against Salmonella

In the heart of this battle against Salmonella, a resounding call to unity echoes through the pages of this chapter. This is not just a fight for survival—it is a fight for the very essence of our humanity. The emotional threads that bind us together become the foundation of our collective strength, as we stand shoulder to shoulder, forging unbreakable bonds against this common enemy.

Imagine the power of a united front—a symphony of voices rising in harmony, each note carrying the weight of compassion, determination, and hope. The emotional resonance of this call to unity reverberates in every heart, for it is through unity that we find the strength to confront the challenges posed by Salmonella.

In this emotional journey, we'll encounter the stories of communities coming together, of individuals reaching out to support one another, and of nations standing as one to combat outbreaks. These emotional connections transcend borders and boundaries, reminding us that the battle against Salmonella is a shared endeavor—one that unites us all as members of the global human family.

As we delve deeper into the emotional power of unity, we must also confront the harsh reality of the barriers that divide us. Language, culture, and geographical distance can seem insurmountable, but within the call to unity lies the power to bridge these gaps and work together for a common cause.

This chapter also celebrates the emotional investment of organizations and governments that rally resources and expertise to fight against Salmonella. Their commitment to public health transcends politics and ideologies, reminding us that the wellbeing of humanity is a cause that unites us all.

The emotional call to unity extends to the dinner table—the very place where the battle against Salmonella begins. As we gather to share meals with loved ones, let us be mindful of the choices we make and the precautions we take to protect each other.

Dear reader, as we embrace the emotional call to unity within this chapter, let us be moved to action. Let compassion guide us in reaching out to those in need, and let determination fuel our efforts to create a safer, healthier world for all.

Let us see past our differences and recognize our shared humanity. The call to unity is an invitation to stand together—stronger, more resilient, and more compassionate. It is through unity that we can triumph over Salmonella, forging a path towards a future where this bacterium no longer casts its shadow on our lives.

Continue with me, as we navigate the emotional symphony of unity. May the stories within this chapter inspire us to be the change we wish to see, as we join hands, hearts, and minds in a powerful chorus—a chorus that will echo through time, heralding our triumph over Salmonella and the dawn of a brighter, safer world for generations to come.

Chapter 12: The Gift of Resilience: Lessons from the Salmonella Struggle

Within the crucible of the Salmonella struggle, an extraordinary gift emerges—the gift of resilience. This chapter explores the emotional transformation that takes place as individuals and communities face adversity head-on, emerging stronger and wiser from the crucible of suffering. Brace yourself, as we bear witness to the indomitable human spirit and the lessons it bestows upon us all.

Imagine a seed buried beneath the soil, facing the darkness and uncertainty of its surroundings. Yet, in that darkness, it finds the strength to push through, reaching towards the light—a symbol of resilience in the face of adversity. In much the same way, the Salmonella struggle shapes individuals, infusing them with the gift of resilience.

In this emotional journey, we'll encounter the stories of survivors—those who have faced the darkness of illness and emerged on the other side. Their emotional transformation is a testament to the human spirit's capacity to endure, to heal, and to embrace life with newfound vigor.

As we delve deeper into the gift of resilience, we must also confront the emotional scars left behind by the Salmonella struggle. The trauma of illness, the fear of recurrence, and the burden of uncertainty—these are the emotional challenges that survivors and their loved ones must navigate.

But amidst the darkness, hope abounds. This chapter celebrates the emotional metamorphosis of survivors, as they find the strength to turn their pain into purpose—to advocate for change, to raise awareness, and to support others facing the same journey.

The gift of resilience extends beyond individuals—it encompasses communities and nations coming together, pledging to do better, to be more proactive in the fight against Salmonella. The emotional impact of this shared determination to protect public health is a force that cannot be underestimated.

Dear reader, as we embrace the emotional gift of resilience within this chapter, let us be moved to introspection. Let us reflect on our own journeys and the emotional struggles we have faced. In the crucible of suffering, we have the opportunity to discover our own resilience—the strength to overcome, to grow, and to thrive.

This chapter is an invitation to learn from the Salmonella struggle—to recognize the gift of resilience within ourselves and others. It is a call to support one another, to offer a helping hand, and to stand united in our collective pursuit of a safer, healthier future.

Continue with me, as we navigate the emotional landscape of resilience. May the stories within this chapter inspire us to embrace the lessons of suffering, to find strength in the face of adversity, and to emerge from the crucible of the Salmonella struggle with hearts alight with hope, compassion, and the unwavering gift of resilience.

Chapter 13: Embracing Hope: A Vision for a Salmonella-Free Future

In the tapestry of our collective struggle against Salmonella, hope emerges as the guiding star—a beacon of light that illuminates the path towards a future free from this relentless threat. This chapter is a tapestry of emotions, woven with threads of optimism, determination, and the unwavering belief that we can shape a world where Salmonella's shadow no longer looms. Prepare to be filled with the emotional charge of hope as we envision a safer, healthier future.

Imagine a world where the specter of Salmonella no longer haunts our meals, our water, or our environment. It is a world where laughter resonates, unburdened by fear, and where the joy of sharing food becomes a celebration of life itself. This vision of a

Salmonella-free future is not a distant dream—it is within our grasp.

In this emotional journey, we'll encounter the stories of individuals and organizations working tirelessly to make this vision a reality. Their emotional investment in the cause of eradicating Salmonella is fueled by hope—a hope that propels them forward, even in the face of daunting challenges.

As we delve deeper into this chapter, we must confront the harsh reality of the work that lies ahead. The battle against Salmonella is not an easy one, but hope shines like a guiding star, leading us towards a brighter tomorrow.

The emotional charge of hope is infectious—it spreads like wildfire, igniting the hearts of individuals, communities, and nations. This chapter celebrates the unity of purpose, the shared determination to protect public health, and the belief that we can overcome any obstacle when we stand together.

The gift of resilience, which we explored in the previous chapter, becomes a powerful catalyst for change. The emotional transformation of survivors, advocates, and professionals becomes the driving force behind a future where Salmonella is no longer a menace.

Dear reader, as we embrace the emotional vision of hope within this chapter, let us be moved to action. Let hope be the spark that ignites our passion, our dedication, and our unwavering commitment to create a safer, healthier world.

This chapter is an invitation to envision a future where Salmonella is but a distant memory. Let us rally behind the emotional call to action—to demand better food safety, to protect our environment, and to support research and innovation that can turn the vision of a Salmonella-free future into a reality.

Continue with me, as we navigate the emotional landscape of hope. May the stories within this chapter inspire us to dream big, to believe in our collective power to effect change, and to forge ahead with hope in our hearts—a hope that will guide us towards the day when Salmonella is vanquished, and the world stands united in triumph against this common enemy.

Chapter 14: A Legacy of Love: Honoring Those Affected by Salmonella

In the wake of the Salmonella struggle, there emerges a poignant legacy—a legacy of love, compassion, and remembrance. This chapter is a heartfelt tribute to those whose lives have been touched by this bacterium, as we honor their memory and draw strength from their stories. Prepare to be moved by the emotional resonance of their legacies—a reminder of the profound impact that Salmonella has had on our lives.

Imagine a garden of memories, each flower representing a life forever touched by Salmonella. Each bloom is a testament to the love shared, the laughter cherished, and the lives forever changed. In this garden of emotions, we find solace, as we honor the resilience of survivors and mourn the loss of those no longer with us.

In this emotional journey, we'll encounter the stories of families who have lost loved ones to Salmonella, their grief palpable in every . Their emotional journey is one of heartbreak and pain, but within their stories lies the power to inspire change—to ensure that no more lives are lost to this preventable bacterium.

As we delve deeper into the legacy of love, we must also confront the harsh reality of the emotional toll that Salmonella takes on families and communities. The aftermath of an outbreak leaves scars that may never fully heal, but within the heartache lies a determination to prevent further suffering.

This chapter is also a tribute to the tireless work of advocates and organizations who have dedicated themselves to honoring the memory of those affected by Salmonella. Their emotional investment in creating awareness, supporting research, and demanding change is a testament to the enduring power of love.

The legacy of love extends to medical professionals and researchers, who carry the weight of responsibility to protect public health. Their emotional commitment to better treatments and prevention becomes a powerful force in the fight against Salmonella.

Dear reader, as we embrace the emotional legacy of love within this chapter, let us be moved to empathy. Let us honor the memory of those affected by Salmonella by standing united in our dedication to prevent further suffering.

This chapter is an invitation to remember—to remember the lives lost, the survivors' resilience, and the love that binds us all together. Let us draw strength from their stories and use it as fuel to continue the fight against Salmonella.

Continue with me, as we navigate the emotional garden of memories. May the stories within this chapter inspire us to act with compassion, to demand accountability, and to create a world where the legacy of love triumphs over the legacy of suffering. Let us carry the memory of those affected by Salmonella in our hearts, and may their legacies be a guiding light on our path towards a safer, healthier future for all.

Chapter 15: A Journey of Hope: Embracing a Salmonella-Free Tomorrow

As we reach the culmination of this emotional journey, we stand on the precipice of a new beginning—a tomorrow free from the grasp of Salmonella. This chapter is a heartfelt ode to hope—a hope that has fueled our quest, transformed our perspectives, and united us in a shared purpose. Prepare to be moved, for within these final pages, we find the emotional crescendo of our journey—a crescendo that heralds the dawn of a new era.

Imagine a world where the specter of Salmonella is vanquished, where food is no longer a source of fear, and where water and nature thrive in harmony. It is a world born from our collective hope—a hope that refuses to be extinguished by challenges and setbacks.

In this emotional journey, we have witnessed the profound impact of Salmonella on individuals, families, and communities. We have explored the resilience of survivors, the dedication of advocates, and the passion of researchers. We have borne witness to the emotional complexities of the struggle, and in doing so, we have become stewards of hope.

As we stand on the threshold of a Salmonella-free tomorrow, we must remember that hope is not a passive state—it is an active force that compels us to action. The emotional call to rise above complacency, to demand change, and to envision a safer world becomes our rallying cry.

This chapter is an invitation to embrace hope as our guiding star—to see beyond the obstacles and envision a future where Salmonella's hold on humanity is but a distant memory. Let us be inspired by the emotional resilience of survivors and advocates, and let their stories be the fuel that propels us forward.

The journey of hope is one of unity, as we recognize that we are not alone in this fight. Our emotional connection to one another and to the cause of safeguarding public health binds us in a shared vision of a better world.

Dear reader, as we embrace the emotional crescendo of hope within this chapter, let us be moved to action. Let hope be the force that drives us to demand accountability, to support research and innovation, and to advocate for a future where Salmonella is no longer a threat.

This chapter is a testament to the power of hope—the power to transform, to heal, and to create lasting change. Let us carry this hope with us, as we step into the unknown of tomorrow, for it is through hope that we can build a future where Salmonella's shadow no longer looms.

Continue with me, as we navigate the emotional landscape of hope. May the stories within this chapter inspire us to be the architects of a Salmonella-free tomorrow—a tomorrow filled with hope, compassion, and the unwavering belief that together, we can triumph over any adversity that comes our way. Let hope be our guiding light, leading us towards a future where health, safety, and love prevail.

Printed in Great Britain
by Amazon

60479878R00047